Too Young to Feel this Old

A Guide to Healthy Aging with Hormones
Stewart Parnacott, CRNA

Contents

1
A Journey to Rediscovering Vitality

As I sat on my porch that fateful Saturday morning, enveloped by the warmth of the Houston sun, little did I know that a simple manila envelope would lead me on a life-changing path toward healthy aging. Exhausted from the demanding responsibilities of my career as a Certified Registered Nurse Anesthetist (CRNA), a nurse practitioner, and a personal trainer, I felt far older than my years would suggest. The boundless energy of my youth seemed like a distant memory, replaced by fatigue and a lack of motivation.

Then, as luck would have it, I crossed paths with a remarkable individual—a chiropractor and fellow CRNA—who introduced me to the fascinating world of bioidentical hormone replacement therapy (BHRT). She had been at the forefront of this revolutionary approach to healthy aging. We connected over similar interests, and in one of our conversations, she shared a book that would forever alter my perspective on aging and vitality—talk about a pivotal moment!

Curious and eager to find a solution to my relentless exhaustion, I began delving into the book's pages, and with each word, a new world of possibilities unfolded before my eyes. I learned about the power of bioidentical hormones—naturally derived compounds that mirror the molecular structure of hormones in the human body. This revelation shattered the notion that only pharmaceutical drugs held the key to effective treatment.

As I read, I couldn't help but notice the parallels between the author's experiences and my own. Symptoms that I had attributed to depression were discussed, and the potential treatments aligned with my own self-diagnosis. My fascination grew as I discovered that the pharmaceutical industry's practice of altering hormones for the purpose of getting a legal patent had led to the development of synthetic drugs, while natural, bioidentical hormones offered a more promising and individualized approach to health.

With each turn of the page, I realized that I wasn't alone in my struggles with aging and vitality. Much like my own, the author's journey had been filled with moments of uncertainty and frustration, ultimately culminating in the discovery of BHRT as a transformative solution. As I reached the end of the book, I began experiencing exceedingly positive changes in my life, mood, and body, and I knew that I couldn't simply keep this knowledge to myself—I had to share it with the world.

This book, "Too Young to Feel This Old: A Guide to Healthy Aging," is the culmination of my own journey and the collective wisdom of medical professionals, researchers, and academics who have explored the realm of bioidentical hormone replacement therapy. Even though I am a medical expert with advanced knowledge, I am not an expert in bioidentical hormones; I am only a few steps ahead of you. I invite you to join me on this transformative path as we explore the science behind healthy aging and the potential of hormone replacement to defy the conventional limitations of time.

As a nurse practitioner and CRNA, I had spent years caring for patients and guiding them on their path to wellness. Yet, in the midst of my demanding career, I had lost sight of my own well-being. The weight of my responsibilities was bearing down on me, and my energy levels plummeted, leaving me feeling like a shadow of my former self. Turning 24, I had anticipated a bright future, but instead, I found myself grappling with unrelenting fatigue and a sense of aging far beyond my years.

This state of perpetual exhaustion was nothing short of disheartening. Fast forward ten years later, and I'm the chief of an anesthesia department at a large hospital in Houston, accustomed to facing challenges head-on and guiding my team through the most demanding situations but still struggling to summon the energy to make it through each day, as I had for the decade prior.

Around the same time, fate would introduce me to an opportunity that would change the trajectory of my life. As my spouse and I explored the possibility of purchasing a business, we came across a hormone replacement clinic for sale in California. The owner, a chiropractor and CRNA like myself, welcomed us with open arms, and our conversations revealed a shared passion for healthcare and healthy aging.

During one of our many discussions, she shared with me a copy of a book that she sends to all her patients to introduce them to the wonders of bioidentical hormone replacement therapy. Intrigued, I began reading the book, and from the first chapter, I found myself captivated. It was as if the author was speaking directly to me, addressing the very symptoms that had weighed me down.

As I immersed myself in the world of bioidentical hormones, I discovered a revelation that defied the traditional approaches to aging. I learned that, unlike synthetic drugs, bioidentical hormones offered a more personalized, natural alternative to restoring vitality and reversing the signs of aging. And with this discovery, I, for the first time in a long time, felt like the missing pieces of the puzzle were finally coming together.

In the following years, my journey of discovery continued, and my passion for healthy aging grew stronger. I sought to understand the scientific foundations behind bioidentical hormone replacement therapy, delving into medical literature and research to uncover the evidence supporting this transformative approach.

As I applied the principles of BHRT to my own life, I experienced a profound change. Newfound energy and a renewed sense of vitality replaced the relentless fatigue that had plagued me for years. The weight I had carried on my shoulders lifted, and I felt like the Stewart of old—motivated, energetic, and ready to tackle whatever challenges came my way. Throughout this transformative journey, I knew with absolute certainty that I had to share the wonders of BHRT.

1.1: A Glimpse of Hope: The Women's Health Initiative Study

Throughout history, the Women's Health Initiative Study (WHI) has played a pivotal role in shaping our understanding of hormone therapy and its impact on health. The WHI explored the effects of hormone replacement in postmenopausal women, leading to important revelations regarding cancer risk and hormone use.

The Women's Health Initiative (WHI) was a groundbreaking study conducted in the early 2000s to investigate the effects of hormone replacement therapy (HRT) in postmenopausal women. Specifically, the study examined the use of estrogen and progestin (Premarin and Provera) in hormone therapy. The WHI found that combined HRT with estrogen and progestin increased the risk of certain health issues, including cardiovascular events and breast cancer, and at the same time, provided some benefits, such as reducing the risk of osteoporotic fractures. As a result of these findings, the use of HRT has become more cautious, and healthcare providers now carefully weigh the potential risks and benefits when considering hormone therapy for menopausal symptom management in women.

I am here to tell you that this WHI study only applies to synthetic hormones created by Big Pharma and does not apply to natural, bioidentical hormones. In fact, bioidentical hormones help those in need of HRT and decrease the risk of cancer, heart disease, and diseases of neurocognitive decline. So why would your local family practice doctor or internal medicine only prescribe you these dangerous synthetic hormones instead of the bioidentical type? We'll explore all of these topics more deeply in the following chapters.

As we traverse the pages of this book, we will delve into the depths of scientific research and explore how the principles of BHRT can provide a rejuvenating alternative for individuals seeking to embrace healthy aging. Together, let us embark on this journey to reclaim our vitality and live life to the fullest, forever young—We're too young to feel this old!

2

Does my doctor hate me? Why would s/he not give me the correct medicine?

Growing up in a small, tight-knit farming town in South Georgia, our access to healthcare was limited. With a median household income of approximately $15,000, preventative medicine was an afterthought, visits to the doctor's office reserved for times of dire illness, and healthcare choices often driven by affordability rather than optimal health.

The media's portrayal of hormone replacement therapy (HRT) has sowed confusion and fear, leading many to believe that hormones are harmful. But avoiding HRT can come with its own set of risks, depriving us of a better, healthier life. The discomfort and pain of an untreated hormone deficiency can be far more taxing than taking the right approach to hormone therapy.

Unfortunately, physicians' hesitancy to prescribe hormones is fueled by conventional medical guidelines—which focus solely on synthetic hormones. They overlook the critical distinction: bioidentical hormones are worlds apart from their synthetic counterparts. While synthetic hormones can pose dangers, bioidentical hormones are safe and offer effective relief.

In the past, I witnessed the fallout of generalized recommendations when the Kaiser organization advised all female patients to discontinue hormones altogether. This blanket approach did a great disservice to these patients. Instead, the focus should have been on discontinuing SYNTHETIC hormones and transitioning to the much safer and biologically identical options, bioidentical hormones.

As I embarked on my journey with bioidentical hormones, it quickly became evident that a deeper understanding of these hormones was essential. The right approach to hormone therapy can be transformative, restoring balance and providing a renewed sense of well-being. So, let's debunk the myths, embrace the power of bioidentical hormones, and reclaim control of our health and happiness. After all, why settle for anything less than the vibrant life we deserve?

2.1: What Happens if I stop hormone replacement altogether?

Medical literature underscores the consequences of long-term hormone deprivation, particularly in women. The alarm shouldn't be the fear of taking hormones but rather the absence of having enough hormones. For example, after a decade of hormone loss, many women may face tooth loss due to diminished mandibular bone support.

Regarding vision, macular degeneration is a severe eye disease that leads to blindness. Remarkably, women on estrogen experience an 80 percent reduction in macular degeneration and vision loss. Discontinuing hormones could mean losing this vital protection.

The benefits of estrogen extend to brain health as well. Women on estrogen for 15 years or more show a significantly lower incidence of Alzheimer's disease. Estrogen's protective effects against dementia are evident and not to be overlooked.

Moreover, starting estrogen therapy at menopause offers a 50 percent reduction in strokes and heart attacks. That's quite a vital benefit to forsake.

Estrogen is also a safeguard against bone loss and osteoporosis, which can have dire consequences. Studies show that 50 percent of women over 65 who suffer hip fractures pass away within two years, underscoring the importance of maintaining bone health.

The implications of hormone loss are widespread, affecting various aspects of a woman's well-being. From brain function and heart health to bone density and cholesterol levels, estrogen plays a pivotal role.

However, unfortunate misinformation persists. Many healthcare providers fail to inform patients of the protection against breast cancer, hair loss, skin changes, and the decline in overall health that follows hormone deprivation.

Progestins, not estrogen or progesterone, carry an increased cancer risk. Women should be wary of medroxyprogesterone (Provera). If hormones were truly harmful, physicians would recommend ovary removal after childbirth. Retaining the ovaries through menopause preserves hormone secretion, leading to better outcomes, including reduced risk of depression, osteoporosis, heart disease, and stroke.

It's not just women who suffer from the effects of hormonal imbalances. Men, too, experience adverse consequences such as decreased libido, muscle loss, and potential prostate issues when hormones are not balanced.

Most doctors' preference for synthetic hormones is a product of their training and the influence of Big Pharma. Bioidentical hormones cannot be patented as they closely resemble those naturally found in the human body. Unfortunately, altering the biomolecular structure of hormones to make them patentable often leads to severe side effects in patients.

This pharmaceutical-driven approach highlights the flaws in our healthcare system, where treating diseases and profiting off of treating those diseases is prioritized over prevention. Bioidentical hormones offer both therapeutic and preventive benefits, but insurance coverage often restricts access to these life-changing therapies. As healthcare professionals, our responsibility is to advocate for better alternatives that prioritize patient well-being over profit-driven practices.

3
Bioidentical Hormones – The Science Unveiled

Once upon a time, in the mystical world of hormones, a battle of epic proportions between the synthetic and the bioidentical raged on. In one corner, standing tall, we have the synthetic hormones concocted by the formidable big pharma companies. Much like a Picasso painting gone awry, these synthetic hormones sport molecular makeups that seem alien to our bodies. Imagine, if you will, trying to fit a square peg into a round hole—quite the mismatch. Don't you think?

And oh, the side effects! These synthetic hormones love playing tricks on us, leaving us with mood swings that could give Shakespeare's dramas a run for their money, bloating, and a whole circus of discomforts. But wait, the plot thickens! Cue the bioidentical hormones—the true stars of our tale. These naturally derived hormone superheroes come armed with a secret weapon, i.e., the perfect molecular match to our body's own hormones.

Picture this bioidentical hormones waltzing into our cells like the smoothest tango on the dance floor. With a seamless fit, they unlock the doors to our well-being, bringing us one step closer to the fountain of youth. Say goodbye to those pesky side effects and welcome a life where harmony reigns supreme. Choosing bioidentical hormone replacement therapy is like sending out an invitation to a joyous celebration of your health and happiness.

But hold on, dear reader, the story doesn't end here. The plot takes an intriguing twist —we are now pondering the age-old question—are hormones helpful or hazardous? It's true; hormones, like all great adventures, have their fair share of complexities. However, the tale takes an uplifting turn when bioidentical hormones come into play.

Unlike their synthetic counterparts, bioidentical hormones come bearing gifts of safety and efficacy. As we delve into the scientific tapestry, we discover that these hormonally gifted superheroes align seamlessly with our natural biology. It's like finding the perfect match on a dating app—when you know, you know. And our bodies know that bioidentical hormones are the real deal, reducing the risk of side effects and steering us towards a smoother, more radiant journey through life.

So, here's the moral of our hormone tale—when you choose bioidentical hormone replacement therapy, you're making a choice for a happier, healthier version of yourself. It's like casting a spell that transforms you into the lead in your own fairytale. Bid farewell to the discomforts of synthetic hormones and step into a world where your well-being takes center stage.

The science behind bioidentical hormones unlocks the true potential of our body's balance, offering a dance of harmony that keeps us moving to the rhythm of life. It's time to embrace the wonders of bioidentical hormones and bask in the joy of living life to its fullest, cheekily and vibrantly. And with that, we leave you with a twinkle in your eye and a newfound zest for life—ready to embark on the next chapter of this delightful journey. The magic of bioidentical hormones awaits, and it's a tale worth telling and living.

3.1: Common Aging Signs and Symptoms – The Age-Defying Battle

Ah, the delightful journey of aging—the gift that keeps on giving! As we gracefully navigate the realms of time, we encounter some charming companions along the way—aging signs and symptoms. Picture them as your personal paparazzi, eager to capture every moment of your life's blockbuster. While they may seem like pesky intruders, fear them not—with the right knowledge and tools, you can give them a run for their money.

1. Pesky Fatigue: The Uninvited Guest Oh, the joys of feeling tired before the day even begins—a tale as old as time! We all know the scene—a yawn-filled morning that stretches into an afternoon of battling fatigue. But have no fear, for bioidentical hormones are here! With their superpowers of

energy restoration, they breathe life into our tired souls. So, bid farewell to the snooze button and welcome back the boundless energy of your youthful days!

2. Hormonal Rollercoaster: The Mood Swing Brigade As we age, hormones love to take us on a rollercoaster ride, leaving us spinning with mood swings that could rival a teacup twirl at Disneyland. But don't let those hormonal daredevils dictate your emotions! Bioidentical hormones are the ultimate mood stabilizers, bringing harmony to your emotional landscape. Bid adieu to those tumultuous emotional voyages and sail through life with a newfound serenity.

3. Cognitive Crossroads: The Brain's Navigation Quest Ah, the curious case of cognitive changes— it feels like the brain is playing hide-and-seek with our memories! But fear not, dear reader, for bioidentical hormones are on a treasure hunt to restore your mental prowess. They arm your brain with the tools it needs to tackle memory lapses and keep your cognitive ship sailing smoothly. With bioidentical hormones as your compass, you'll be navigating through life's challenges with wit and clarity.

4. The Sluggish Metabolism: The Unwanted Stowaway Say hello to the not-so-welcome stowaway—sluggish metabolism! As we age, pesky extra pounds, sans invitation, seem too eager to take up residence all over our bodies. But hark, there's hope on the horizon! Bioidentical hormones are the ultimate metabolism boosters.

They'll rev up your body's engine and help you shed that unwanted weight. So, wave goodbye to those unwelcome pounds and embrace the vitality of your youthful days.

5. Beauty Battle Royale: The Skin's Secret Weapon Ah, the secrets of youthful skin—the enigma that has intrigued the ages. But guess what? Bioidentical hormones are here to unlock the beauty code! With their magical-like touch, they restore your skin's radiant glow by reducing the pesky wrinkles and blemishes. So, say farewell to the skincare aisle and welcome the age-defying magic of bioidentical hormones.

6. Energy Depletion: The Lethargy Dilemma Ever feel like your energy bar is running on empty? We've all been there—cue the afternoon slump that lingers well into the evening. Well, fret not — bioidentical hormones are ready to recharge your energy reserves. They act as your body's personal Energizer Bunny, keeping you going and going and going. Say goodbye to the lethargy and hello to the boundless energy of your youthful days!

7. The Sleep Saga: The Dreamland Challenge Ah, the elusive quest for a good night's sleep—a tale as old as time. But fear not, for bioidentical hormones are your sleep's fairy godmothers, waving their wands to grant you peaceful slumber. Say farewell to those sleepless nights and welcome the sweet embrace of dreamland.

8. The Mighty Libido: The Passionate Flame Our once fiery passion may seem like a flickering candle as we age. But lo and behold, bioidentical

hormones are the spark that reignites the flame of desire. Say hello to a rekindled passion and bid adieu to the cooling embers.

So, dear reader, as we journey through the common aging signs and symptoms, remember this—you hold the key to unlocking the secrets of youthful vitality. Armed with the magic of bioidentical hormones, you can dance through life with a cheeky grin and the confidence of a true age-defying warrior. Embrace the journey, the science, and the marvels of bioidentical hormones—the elixir of youth awaits you!

3.2: Empowering Your Immune System – Unleashing Your Inner Superhero

Does your once mighty immune system, aka the tall-standing, powerful shield against invaders, no longer seem indestructible? Well, dear reader, even the mightiest shield inevitably shows signs of wear and tear as time marches on. As the years pass, the once indomitable fortress of your immune system may begin to show chinks in its armor, leaving you susceptible to unwelcome guests like colds and infections. Fortunately, the bioidentical hormone brigade is here to the rescue!

Imagine this—you don the cape and become the superhero of your immune system, ready to vanquish those pesky invaders. With bioidentical hormones as your trusty sidekicks, your immune system undergoes a renaissance—emerging stronger, fiercer, and more resilient than ever before. And just like that, you forget dull days of sniffles and coughs and welcome a world where your immune fortress stands tall, repelling invaders like an impenetrable shield.

Naturally, you might wonder, "How do these bioidentical hormones work their magic?" Worry not. Science is here to unravel the secrets. Bioidentical hormones, born from natural sources, are the perfect fit for your body's receptors. They slide into action, signaling your immune cells to rise and defend. It's like a superhero team-up. Imagine the Avengers, in the hormone world, working in perfect harmony to keep you strong and healthy.

Now, let's get into the perks of having a well-empowered immune system. Saying goodbye to those never-ending colds and infections that once seemed inevitable is but one of the many perks of a well-empowered immune system. With bioidentical hormones as your loyal allies, you will be poised to take on anything life throws your way. So, suit up, immune superhero! Your days of vulnerability are behind you—a world of strength and resilience awaits.

Oh, and of course, let's not forget the cheeky humor—the secret weapon of any age-defying superhero! Picture this: your immune system, donning a cape and a cheeky grin, ready to conquer those invaders with a twinkle in its eye. It's the kind of superhero story that Marvel could only dream of—a tale of rejuvenation and triumph.

A strong immune system is not just about defense but also about balance. Your bioidentical hormone allies help ensure that your immune system dances in perfect harmony, avoiding both underactivity and overactivity. No more immune system parties gone awry, leading to allergies and autoimmune woes. Instead, your immune system becomes the maestro of balance, conducting its symphony of protection with finesse.

So, dear reader, embrace the power of bioidentical hormones—the age-defying elixirs that awaken the superhero within. Empower your immune system, let it soar to new heights, and bid farewell to the days of vulnerability. With bioidentical hormones by your side, you're the captain of your immune fortress—a force to be reckoned with, a true age-defying superhero.

3.3: Unraveling the Cancer Connection - Shedding Light on Hope

The shadow of cancer—a chilling specter that looms over our lives, casting an unsettling sense of fear and uncertainty. But hold on tight, dear reader, for in the face of darkness, there shines a ray of hope—a beacon of light that promises a brighter tomorrow. Prepare yourself for a revelation that defies expectations—the brave souls who embraced bioidentical hormone replacement therapy reaped more than just the rewards of ageless vitality. They were granted a remarkable gift—a decreased risk of certain cancers, including the dreaded breast cancer. Yes, you read that right! The magic of bioidentical hormones extends far beyond defying one's age—it's a formidable ally in the battle against life-altering diseases.

Now, let's delve into the science that unveils the wondrous connection between bioidentical hormones and cancer protection. Think of it as a symphony of biochemical harmony—a delicate dance between hormones and receptors, orchestrating a melody of cancer prevention, bioidentical hormones being the virtuoso. Because bioidentical hormones are born from natural sources, they are perfectly attuned to our body's needs. So, they gracefully step in and conduct a symphony that keeps cancer at bay.

In case you are wondering, "How can hormones be the champions of cancer protection?" Let me share the secret—their natural, perfect molecular fit. It's like a lock and key mechanism—bioidentical hormones fit seamlessly into the receptors, unlocking a cascade of protective responses. No artificial tweaks—no unwanted side effects—just a beautiful dance of balance that keeps the enemy at bay.

With that, let's raise our glasses to the hormones that have our backs—the true heroes in our fight against aging and cancer. Bioidentical hormones—the valiant guardians of our well-being that defy expectations and bring hope where there once was fear.

With their help, we stand tall, daring to live life to the fullest, unshackled by the dark cloud of cancer's shadow.

But before we conclude, let's add a dash of humor to our celebration of science and triumph. Try picturing hormones, dancing joyfully in the spotlight, dressed in capes of courage and humor. They may be tiny molecules, but their impact on our lives is immeasurable. They say laughter is the best medicine, but with bioidentical hormones, we have an unbeatable duo—laughter and protection, the ultimate elixir of life.

So, dear reader, as we bask in the light of this newfound hope, let's remember the power we hold—the power to embrace bioidentical hormones, the age-defying warriors that grant us vitality, strength, and the shield against cancer's grip. Let us stand together, united in our fight for a life of boundless joy and freedom from fear. With bioidentical hormones as our steadfast companions, the future shines bright, a testament to the triumph of science, humor, and the indomitable human spirit.

4
Understanding the Aging Process

Ah, aging—the inevitable journey we must all embark on, like seasoned travelers wandering through the enigmatic landscapes of time. Our bodies, akin to complex works of art, undergo a symphony of changes as we navigate the intricacies of life. Welcome to the fascinating realm of the science of aging, where we delve into the very essence of what makes us age and how we can rewrite the rules of this grand voyage.

Now, before we dive into the science behind the curtain of time, let's take a moment to appreciate the marvel of individuality. While aging is a universal concept, the pace at which it touches our lives is as unique as a fingerprint. Blame it on our genes, lifestyle choices, perhaps even the whims of Mother Nature—these factors weave a tapestry of time that's entirely our own.

As we tread gracefully through the years, our hormonal landscape begins to shift, much like the ever-changing seasons. Picture this: A hormone party that's been going strong since the day we were born is now slowing down its tempo. Yes, my dear readers, the hormones that once danced with youthful exuberance are taking a well-deserved break, and this hiatus comes with a twist.

As these hormonal shifts unfold, they bring along a fascinating array of signs and symptoms, putting even the greatest detective's skills to the test. Do you get pesky common colds that seemingly linger longer than unwelcome guests at a party? If you answered Yes, I hate to break it to you, but they might just be a product of our hormonal drumline playing a different tune. And let's not forget the sly cancer risk that tries to tip the scales in its favor.

But fret not, for in this realm of science and discovery, we have, at our fingertips, a magical solution, i.e., bioidentical hormones. These hormone marvels, born from nature's finest creations, stand ready to swing the pendulum back in our favor. With the help of these hormonally gifted superheroes, we can combat the signs of aging and embrace a new era of vitality.

So, buckle up, dear reader, as we journey through the secrets of time. Prepare to be enchanted by the science that unlocks the mysteries of aging and the transformative power of bioidentical hormones. Here, we blend the wisdom of ages with the wonders of science, all while embracing the charm of cheeky humor. Get ready to challenge the norms of aging, armed with the magic of knowledge and the resilience of a curious mind. In this voyage, we will uncover the truth behind the ticking clock and dance our way to a future filled with vitality and joy.

4.1: Hormones as the Age Gauge: The Role of DHEA

As I embarked on my journey through graduate school at age 23, I felt and was a force to be reckoned with. I was full of energy and ready to conquer the world, or at least my career. But by age 24, things began to change. The energy that once fueled me was dwindling, my libido took an unexpected detour, and my muscles seemed to have gone on vacation without me. To top it all off, the stress of my studies and working in the operating room felt like heavy weights dragging me down. As the years passed, I found myself feeling even worse. The fatigue became overwhelming, and the once fiery passion in the bedroom became nothing but a flicker. I searched for answers, wondering if it was depression creeping in, but I was hesitant to turn to antidepressants, fearing they might further dampen my already diminishing sex drive.

Then, like a beacon of hope, I discovered bioidentical hormones—a cure I never knew existed but one that would prove to be a savior. With these hormones, my sex life got a second wind, and I felt a renewed excitement for life. Not only did I regain my lost energy and sexual prowess, but the weight gain that had stealthily crept on over the past decade began to melt away. It was like witnessing a transformation before my eyes. As the pounds vanished, my skin seemed to glow with newfound radiance, and my muscles started to regain their long-lost definition.

I regained my ability to go for multiple rounds in the bedroom, reigniting the passion that had been waning for so long. It was like a revelation that brought back the vitality and vigor I thought were forever lost. It's incredible how these tiny, cheeky hormones not only saved my sex life but also restored my overall well-being, making me feel like a new person altogether. Sometimes, all it takes is a little cheekiness to uncover the secret to reclaiming the life we thought was slipping through our fingers.

4.2: DHEA: One of the Real Superstars

As a seasoned healthcare professional, I can attest to the remarkable impact of hormone replacement therapy (HRT) in transforming lives and rejuvenating vitality. HRT is not a cure for mortality, but it extends the canvas of life with vibrancy, excitement, and fulfillment. It empowers individuals to age gracefully, free from the clutches of the physical and mental decline that have plagued previous generations. The magic of bioidentical hormones, particularly DHEA, breathes life into worn-out bodies, alleviating unimaginable joint pain, nerve discomfort, and more. In this chapter, we embark on a journey through the realm of DHEA, uncovering its pivotal role in sustaining health, resilience, and longevity.

1. The Dance of Hormones: The Adrenal Gland's Decline - As we journey through the passage of time, the adrenal gland's zona reticularis, the fountainhead of DHEA production, undergoes atrophy. By the time we reach 80, our DHEA levels plummet to a mere 10 to 20 percent of what we once had in our vibrant mid-20s. This hormonal nosedive profoundly impacts not only gender health but also the immune system, heart health, and susceptibility to cancer and autoimmune disorders. Several reputable medical journals have extensively documented the significance of DHEA in thwarting diabetes, heart disease, and cancer. High DHEA levels signify increased longevity, while low levels predict early mortality. Embracing the benefits of DHEA is pivotal for well-being.

2. DHEA: The Guardian of Health and Youth - In 'the grand orchestra of hormones,' DHEA deserves a standing ovation. This hormone has proven to be a potent inhibitor of disease, a guardian of youth, and a sustainer of health. The immune system, often the culprit behind disorders like lupus and osteoporosis, faces a formidable ally in DHEA. Early supplementation with DHEA prevents the shrinkage of the thymus gland, halting immunosenescence before it takes root. The path to longevity lies in prevention, and DHEA leads the way.

3. The Balancing Act: DHEA and Cortisol - In the intricate dance of hormones, DHEA and cortisol play an intertwined duet. When cortisol rises in

response to stress, DHEA counters its effects. Too much stress leads to excessive cortisol production, which suppresses DHEA levels, thus accelerating the aging process. Maintaining youthful DHEA levels helps manage cortisol, safeguarding against detrimental effects on the heart and overall health. My personal experience with hormone replacement, specifically DHEA, attests to its ability to tune up the brain and enhance cognitive function under stress.

4. The Elixir of Wellness: DHEA's Cancer-Fighting Potential - DHEA showcases its versatility as a hormone capable of converting to both estradiol and testosterone. This transformation leads to a decrease in visceral fat, mitigating the risk of diabetes and heart disease. By maintaining DHEA at youthful levels, the body's systems harmonize and work in unison, guarding against the development of certain cancers and promoting overall well-being. The ripple effect of balanced hormones reverberates through the body, fostering vitality and health.

5. Illuminating Insulin Sensitivity: DHEA's Impact on Diabetes - While advocating for healthy lifestyle choices is essential, sometimes it is not enough to combat the ravages of time. DHEA's benefits extend to reducing insulin resistance and improving insulin sensitivity. Recent research in the Journal of Lipid Research reveals DHEA's antiatherogenic effects, safeguarding against the accumulation of arterial plaques and promoting

heart health by balancing HDL and LDL lipoproteins.

In conclusion, DHEA emerges as the elixir of vitality, infusing life with the vibrancy of youth and the fortitude of health. Bioidentical hormone replacement therapy opens doors to a world where graceful aging is not simply a dream but a reality to embrace. As a healthcare professional, I celebrate the wonders of hormonal harmony, where DHEA orchestrates a symphony of well-being, resonating through the body and mind. The pathway to enduring vitality and a fulfilling life lies in the balance of hormones, and DHEA shines as a guiding light in this symphony of health. As we unravel the beauty of bioidentical hormones, the promise of a life lived to the fullest awaits, with DHEA leading the way to the fountain of vitality and resilience.

5
Progesterone: Nature's Partner in the Aging Symphony – Hormonal Harmony and the Elixir of Youth

Numerous women find relief from their PMS symptoms when incorporating progesterone into their regimen. Even women who are in menopause or are postmenopausal find symptomatic relief with the incorporation of progesterone. In the early stages of hormone replacement therapy, it was not widely acknowledged that two pivotal ovarian hormones, estrogen and progesterone, govern the female body and sexuality.

Without progesterone's balancing effects, estrogen can turn into a counterproductive element for the uterus. Conditions such as uterine or endometrial cancer often result from excessive estrogen stimulation of uterine tissue. Younger women are less susceptible due to their ample progesterone production, which naturally balances estrogen. Post-menopause, progesterone production diminishes, putting women at risk of estrogen dominance or excessive stimulation of estrogen receptor sites. Incorporation of natural bioidentical progesterone can downregulate these receptor sites, inhibiting excessive estrogen stimulation in the breast and uterus while providing other beneficial effects. Optimally, all hormones should be replaced to pre-menopausal levels for their overall benefits.

Progesterone, synthesized in the corpus luteum, adrenal glands, and placenta during pregnancy, becomes less abundant as women enter their 30s. Post-menopause, progesterone levels plummet nearly to zero, and without proper progesterone levels, women may experience hot flashes, night sweats, and insomnia. A common sentiment among women undergoing bioidentical hormone replacement therapy with estrogen and progesterone is that they regain a sense of vitality. In some instances where women perceive their antidepressants as ineffective, the root cause might be a hormone deficiency rather than depression, thus offering a path to reclaiming their lives.

Menopausal symptoms, including emotional instability, headaches, and mood swings, can be alleviated with natural progesterone. Progesterone's therapeutic impact extends beyond its role as a tranquilizer, also encompassing its potential as an antidepressant, natural pain reliever, and effective remedy for premenstrual syndrome (PMS). Many healthcare providers prescribe antidepressants for PMS, which often only yield marginal improvement.

During the menopausal transition, women navigate significant life changes. Children leave for college or get married, marital dynamics shift, and couples adapt to new surroundings. Amidst these changes, women juggle work, family, and personal time. Menopause can tip this delicate balance, causing depression. Progesterone's innate calming effect can help redirect menopausal depression, enabling women to wake up rejuvenated for the new day.

5.1: Sleep's Influence on Well-being

The correlation between sleep duration and mood and health is undeniable. Sleep loss during menopause is a major disruptive factor. Lethargy, daytime apathy, and nocturnal anxiety are common complaints. A study from the early 2000s revealed that women taking natural progesterone experienced significantly improved sleep compared to those on the synthetic hormone Provera®. This difference is due to the tranquilizing effects of progesterone, which contrasts with Provera's® depressive impact.

The body's response to the sudden shift and decline of hormones is astonishing. Progesterone deficiency can trigger both minor and major complications.

5.2: Guarding Heart Health

Heart disease ranks as the leading cause of death in women. Regrettably, Provera® has been shown to counteract some of estrogen's heart-protective benefits, tarnishing the reputation of natural progesterone. Even so, synthetic hormones like

Provera® are widely prescribed, whereas natural progesterone remains largely overlooked. Provera's® detrimental effects prompted research into the heart-protective qualities of natural bioidentical progesterone, yielding promising results. Now, let me clear up a misconception—Provera® is not progesterone. The two have distinct molecular structures. Bioidentical progesterone synergizes with estrogen, maintaining youthful heart function. Conversely, Provera® antagonizes estrogen, negating its heart benefits.

5.3: Progesterone's Role in Bone Health

Progesterone enhances estrogen's impact on bone health, particularly in promoting the function of osteoblasts that aid in building new bone. Since bones undergo continuous construction and deconstruction, progesterone's role in this balance is vital.

5.4: Synergy between Estrogen and Progesterone

Synergy means that the effect of one item is made stronger by the addition of another. Our Math teachers taught us that $1 + 1 = 2$, right? Well, here's a plot twist. In this scenario, estrogen is (1) and progesterone is (1). When combining the two hormones, $1 + 1 \geq 3$. Estrogen and progesterone synergize, creating an effect that's greater than their individual contributions. Both hormones protect eyes, teeth, heart, bones, skin, vaginal tissue, and lipids. Losing these hormones equates to losing their protective benefits.

5.5: Addressing Myths and Misconceptions

Dispelling myths is essential, and one common misconception is that progesterone is unnecessary for women without a uterus. However, progesterone offers benefits to various organs beyond uterine protection. Whether or not women have a uterus, they still have progesterone receptors in their bodies. Therefore, progesterone remains a necessity at any age for all women.

Many healthcare providers incorrectly believed that progesterone solely safeguarded the uterus. This myth poses a hurdle to effective hormone replacement therapy.

For women without a uterus, the need for progesterone is evident. The body's many progesterone receptors respond positively to its presence.

Lack of progesterone can lead to age-related diseases, similar to estrogen deficiency. Optimal levels of natural progesterone maintain proper bone density, heart health, lower cholesterol, quality of life, contentment, enhancement of estrogen's benefits, protection against breast and uterine cancer, prevention of vaginal atrophy, and relief from PMS. Replacing hormones with their natural counterparts is the key to achieving complete health.

5.6: Distinguishing Between Synthetic and Natural Hormones

The benefits of estrogen and progesterone in averting age-related ailments are well-established. However, most prescriptions are for synthetic forms, such as Premarin® and Provera®, which have different structures from human hormones and thus function differently. Provera®, in fact, is made from the urine of pregnant mares. Yes, that's right: your doctor prescribed you horse hormones. Approximately ten different hormones are isolated from the horse urine to make Provera®, and your body naturally recognizes this treatment as being very foreign, hence the terrible side effects.

Synthetic hormones contribute to adverse side effects, whereas natural hormones offer all benefits without the drawbacks.

Medical advancements prolong our lifespan, but the goal is also to enhance its quality. Embracing natural progesterone and estrogen can safeguard against heart disease, stroke, cancer, osteoporosis, and Alzheimer's. These hormones improve skin, mood, sex life, and self-image, allowing the years from 30 to 130 to be the best of our years.

6
Estrogen: The Genesis of Hormone Replacement – Navigating the Hormonal Crossroads of Aging Heart Health

Estrogen, the very hormone that pioneered total hormone replacement therapy, has faced undeserved criticism of late. This unjust perception has led countless women to suffer needlessly, swayed by sensationalism. Distilling accurate information free from hyperbole into the minds of women and their healthcare providers has become a challenge. In the spring of 2003, the Women's Health Initiative study spotlighted increased risks of heart attacks, strokes, breast cancer, and dementia. Women nationwide discontinued hormone use, while doctors remained unsure, failing to offer alternatives. This chapter delves into the concept of bioidentical hormones, and as you'll discover within the chapter, it's a concept that holds remarkable potential.

Menopause's challenges first thrust hormone replacement therapy into the limelight. For almost 60 years, doctors prescribed estrogen to alleviate menopausal symptoms like hot flashes, vaginal dryness, concentration problems, anxiety, and insomnia. The results were astonishing, with some women continuing estrogen even post-menopause. These women enjoyed better lives, looking and feeling improved. Beyond cosmetic perks—lustrous hair, smoother skin, and toned muscles, their estrogen-mitigated osteoporosis, heart disease, and colon cancer risks decreased. These unforeseen benefits drove a closer examination of hormones' role in health and aging.

6.1: Estrogen as a Disease Fighter

Why embrace estrogen? Estrogen guards against or mitigates heart disease, stroke, high cholesterol, Alzheimer's disease, memory loss, menopausal symptoms, osteoporosis, urinary tract atrophy, skin atrophy, depression, and mood swings.

For centuries, people saw menopause as a mere transition into old age. However, it's a pivotal phase that can transform into a vibrant second adulthood. Women now live 30 to 40 years beyond menopause, a period deserving of critical attention. To maximize post-menopausal years, resources to enhance this stage are essential. Estrogen and progesterone offer an answer. They've proven not only effective but surpassed expectations at infusing renewed vitality.

Estrogen, an essential hormone, tackles menopausal discomfort while nurturing a youthful internal environment. Its replacement is a safe, effective countermeasure against aging's complexities.

Natural bioidentical estrogen bolsters bone health, averts heart issues, and safeguards against Alzheimer's. It's a shield against the ailments age can bring.

This chapter's aim is to magnify bioidentical estrogen's undeniable benefits to women. The rewards far outweigh the risks. The main risk lies in under-replacing estrogen. The risks noted in the Women's Health Initiative trial stemmed from synthetic estrogen. Bioidentical estrogen usage has not demonstrated these risks. The distinctions between natural and synthetic forms of estrogen and progesterone will become apparent as we explore the benefits and risks of both. Women deserve lives free from bone loss, heart ailments, and Alzheimer's. Natural estrogen's power, I stand by, offering robust support for the female body. Post-reading, I hope you'll comprehend how natural hormones nurture beyond middle age. In addressing the Women's Health Initiative and its findings, clarity will emerge about the differences between synthetic and natural estrogen—a distinction vital for optimal health.

Consider this book your resource as a patient or healthcare provider. It's designed to untangle the hype spun from skewed studies, helping you embrace estrogen replacement without fear. Enjoy a healthier, happier life. Since the Women's Health Initiative's publication, subsequent studies have demonstrated that estrogen, be it synthetic or natural, poses no stroke or heart disease risk when initiated soon after menopause. Estrogen alone predicted protection against both heart disease and strokes. If estrogen were harmful, we would get our ovaries removed at 30. Yet, we strive to preserve ovaries during hysterectomies due to negative symptoms and subsequent heart and bone issues. Studies reveal estrogen and other hormones are so beneficial that ovarian function should endure as long as possible. Don't dread estrogen; dread its loss.

The Women's Health Initiative stirred panic. Approximately 50% of hormone users discontinued treatment, often without consulting doctors or understanding the study. Many physicians misunderstood the methodology, advising cessation without alternatives. Women sought relief from symptoms like hot flashes, mood swings, and depression, returning to risky synthetic hormones. This choice ensued when a safe, natural alternative existed.

This panic's consequence is unfortunate—women missing out on estrogen's incredible benefits. This choice arises from fear and perceived risk. While fear is natural, it's important to note that the risks were minimal. The increased breast cancer risk was less than one person per thousand, and it arose solely from Premarin and Provera's combination. The Women's Health Initiative showed no increased breast cancer risk with estrogen alone—the study focused on synthetic estrogen, Premarin, and progestin, Provera.

Before we proceed, please allow me to reiterate that Provera is not progesterone. Okay, now let's get back to The Women's Health Initiative study—the study involved different drug combinations, but the increased breast cancer risk emerged from the Premarin and Provera arm. The risk was detected early and linked to Provera. It was in no way attributed to estrogen. Synthetic progestins, like Provera, have raised cancer risk before. Premarin contains 10 synthetic versions of estrogens found in the human body. Recent studies linked an 8-fold cancer risk increase with Provera addition. Provera increases breast cancer risk. Despite the Women's Health Initiative, the blame for increased breast cancer risk still falls on estrogen. The estrogen-only arm only demonstrated a slightly increased stroke risk in older women aged 65 and above who initiated therapy after 65. However, this wasn't seen in younger women under 60 or in women starting within five years of menopause. Numerous studies confirm estrogen's benefits in heart attack, heart disease, and stroke prevention, especially in younger women. Premarin, however, increases clotting in heart, leg, and lung arteries and veins. A recent JAMA study confirmed this, finding natural estrogen did not increase clotting risk. Increased clotting was linked to the horse estrogen in Premarin.

Regrettably, the media misrepresented the Women's Health Initiative findings, indicting all hormone therapy. Synthetic progestin Provera and horse estrogen Premarin are the culprits, not natural estrogen or progesterone.

6.2: Estrogen in the Headlines

Let's delve into the distinct nature of hormones, ensuring clarity in definitions. The terms "natural" and "synthetic" are often heard, evoking questions of their true essence. My goal is to dispel any misperceptions that may exist. Many doctors incorrectly perceive hormones as uniform. Some denounce natural hormones as valueless, advocating medicinal alternatives. Both notions are misguided.

When I refer to "natural estrogen replacement," "natural progesterone replacement," or the combination of both as "natural hormone replacement," I'm speaking of bioidentical hormones. These match our body's natural hormone composition. The term "natural" has been loosely applied. Some assume it denotes plant-derived products, but this isn't entirely accurate. Many plant-based foods contain phytoestrogens, resembling estrogen, but far weaker—about 1 to 2% of human estrogen potency. These differ from physician-prescribed, pharmacy-compounded natural hormones, which are identical to our body's hormones. Synthetic hormones, like conjugated equine estrogens derived from pregnant mares' urine (Premarin), are commonly used but differ significantly from human hormones, yielding adverse effects not seen with our own hormones.

Bioidentical hormones are molecularly identical to human hormones and sourced from natural plants. Their chemical congruence makes them natural to the body. The body recognizes them as akin to its own production. They are truly a precise fit tailored for your biology.

Why the persistence of synthetic alternatives? A blend of ignorance and cost contributes. Natural supplements and bioidentical hormones lack patentability, reducing pharmaceutical interest. Pharmaceutical companies favor patentable drugs for profit. Much physician education comes from drug companies, leading to a scarcity of knowledge about bioidentical hormones. These hormones are often not marketed by brand names, requiring proficient healthcare providers to ensure correct prescriptions and proper blood levels—proper hormone absorption and balanced dosages are paramount for success.

6.3: Estrogen as a Menopausal Matchup

Synthetic hormones initially garnered praise for alleviating menopausal symptoms. Yet, long-term studies reveal their harmful effects. Women intolerant of synthetic hormones endure side effects such as breast pain, bleeding, acne, and mood swings. Synthetic hormones' non-identity with the body leads to abnormal metabolites and cancer risks. Natural hormones perfectly match the body, fostering wellness.

Estrogen, a prominent female hormone produced in ovaries and adrenal glands, elevates cardiovascular health, bone integrity, and vessel elasticity. The three types of estrogen—estrone, estradiol, and estriol—work in harmony, safeguarding women throughout life. Estradiol dominates reproductive years, while estrone prevails post-menopause. Estriol, a weaker estrogenic derivative, contributes to hormonal balance.

Beyond easing menopausal blues, estrogen holds further benefits. It counters vaginal dryness and urinary infections, nourishing intimate relationships. It revitalizes skin, staving off age-related changes. Women transitioning into menopause experience discomfort like hot flashes, mood shifts, and skin changes. Post-menopausal symptoms such as cardiovascular risks, osteoporosis, and Alzheimer's can ensue. Estrogen supplementation eradicates these concerns, ensuring quality of life beyond early menopause.

Hot flashes, marked by sudden warmth and excessive sweating, plague 75% of menopausal women. These jolts, attributed to estrogen shortage, disrupt lives. Estrogen supplementation quickly restores composure, positively impacting well-being.

Irregular menstruation is another hallmark of menopause, often aligning with perimenopause's hormone fluctuations.

Mood swings, arising from estrogen's interaction with beta-endorphins, alter perceptions and reactions. Estrogen therapy improves emotional balance and mental health. Vaginal dryness and atrophy, attributed to estrogen receptor loss, disrupt intimacy. Estrogen therapy rejuvenates the genito-urinary tract, enhancing lubrication and reducing infections.

Skin aging is often evident during menopause, characterized by dryness, thinning, and wrinkles. Estrogen, however, bolsters collagen production, supporting hydration and firmness. Women needn't exhaust their finances on cosmetics; estrogen offers a natural solution.

6.4: Estrogen Going Above and Beyond

Estrogen's influence extends beyond comfort; it's pivotal for bone health. After menopause, declining estrogen leads to rapid bone mass loss. Estradiol's significance in bone formation is underscored by its receptor sites within the skeletal structure. Estrogen also facilitates calcium utilization, which is crucial for healthy bones. It's a clear-cut advocate for osteoporosis prevention.

Understanding estrogen's roles enhances our grasp of the aging process and its implications. Through hormone replacement, we can break the chain of aging events, all while thwarting osteoporosis, heart disease, and Alzheimer's. Let's unravel the science.

6.5: Optimizing Hormones for Brain Health

As our understanding of hormones deepens, so does ongoing research continue to unveil the potential benefits of hormone replacement therapy, shedding light on the connection between hormonal balance and brain health. For instance, while estrogen therapy wasn't originally intended as a preventative measure for dementia, recent studies have uncovered remarkable outcomes. Quite often, women who embarked on estrogen therapy reported a noticeable enhancement in memory along with improvement in mood and overall well-being. This phenomenon goes beyond merely alleviating menopause symptoms; rigorous medical investigations have consistently demonstrated that estrogen supplementation positively impacts cognitive function and memory.

It's intriguing to note that some women, previously untouched by depression, encounter a sudden shift in mood during menopause. This response is unsurprising, considering that estrogen plays a role in stabilizing mood. While pharmaceuticals like Prozac and Zoloft are, in essence, designed to mimic optimal estrogen levels, it's important to highlight that estrogen in itself has been a natural mood enhancer.

Many of my patients have witnessed an uplifted outlook and improved emotional balance while on estrogen therapy. In fact, various studies have validated these claims by illustrating estrogen's profound effects on memory, learning, and overall mental acuity.

Considering that women constitute a significant portion of the population over 85 years old, researchers have begun delving into how estrogen might mitigate the risk of Alzheimer's disease—a neurodegenerative condition characterized by the loss of neurons, particularly in areas associated with memory and learning. Interestingly, Alzheimer's progression involves the deposition of beta-amyloid protein and neurofibrillary tangling, ultimately leading to neuron destruction. Estrogen's demonstrated ability to prevent such damage and thwart the onset of Alzheimer's is both promising and groundbreaking.

Beyond Alzheimer's, estrogen's positive effects on mental function and cognition extend to women without the disease. Estrogen appears to not only shield against the underlying pathologies that trigger Alzheimer's but also counteracts the routine memory decline that accompanies aging. The potential to avert Alzheimer's is a significant breakthrough and an opportunity for women to enhance their quality of life in later years.

6.6: The Misunderstood Relationship with Breast Cancer

Estrogen has faced some unwarranted criticism, particularly after flawed reporting during the Women's Health Initiative (WHI). This misinformation has led to unfounded fears of estrogen causing breast cancer. While certain headlines perpetuate this narrative, it's crucial to clarify that the estrogen-only arm of the study demonstrated a decrease in breast cancer incidence. Only when combined with progestin did the risk increase. The truth is that estrogen alone does not cause cancer. It's the addition of progestin that poses a potential risk. Regrettably, the nuanced details of the study often get lost, fueling unnecessary alarm.

The minimal increased risk of breast cancer when using Premarin and progestin is a statistic often overshadowed by sensationalism. It's worth noting that heart disease and stroke, constituting 60% of women's mortality, significantly surpass the risk of breast cancer. However, the spotlight remains on breast cancer, inadvertently diverting attention from the detrimental consequences of estrogen loss, such as heart disease and bone deterioration.

The WHI trials validated that estrogen alone does not heighten the risk of cancer or heart disease. The positive effects of estrogen on heart health are incontestable; it's an unequivocal life-saver. Yet, the focus often remains on the specter of breast cancer rather than acknowledging the harm caused by estrogen deficiency.

6.7: Dispelling Misconceptions and Embracing the Benefits

Breast cancer fears have obscured estrogen's true potential. While headlines emphasize the negative, it's crucial to recognize that estrogen offers a dynamic range of short-term and long-term benefits. Many women fail to acknowledge the heart-saving and cancer-protective advantages due to overblown concerns. In a study, only 35% of women were aware of the link between menopause and heart disease, highlighting the widespread lack of awareness regarding women's health risks.

Addressing these concerns requires a balanced perspective. While there's a slight risk of breast cancer with progestin, estrogen alone is not associated with such risk. On the other hand, without estrogen, risks of heart disease, osteoporosis, Alzheimer's, and colon cancer loom large. Women and their healthcare providers must comprehend these intricacies and weigh the potential benefits against the risks.

It's encouraging that studies are increasingly suggesting that women who survived breast cancer need not forego estrogen's benefits. Over 60 studies indicate that estrogen is safe when administered five years after initial breast cancer treatment. Importantly, no increased recurrence risk has been observed. In fact, estrogen use has been linked to decreased recurrences, lower heart disease risk, and improved survival rates.

It's time to put the spotlight back on estrogen's life-saving potential, focusing on evidence rather than fear. By offering comprehensive education and encouraging informed decisions, healthcare providers can empower women to make choices that enhance their well-being. Estrogen deficiency should not undermine the quality of a woman's life. This book aims to provide clarity and guidance, ensuring women can make the best decisions for their health.

Evidently, estrogen plays a pivotal role in maintaining heart health, preserving bone density, enhancing cognitive function, and elevating emotional well-being in the aging population. The goal is not just to extend life but to improve its quality, and estrogen can be a powerful tool in achieving that goal.

7
Estrogen and Progesterone: Demystifying the Cancer Connection – Unraveling the Hormonal Ties to Cancer Risk

Welcome, dear reader, to a simplified exploration of one of the most intriguing and complex relationships in the realm of hormones—the link between estrogen, progesterone, and cancer risk. As a healthcare professional, I am delighted to take you on this journey of demystifying the cancer connection and shedding light on the intricate hormonal ties that may influence cancer risk for both men and women.

7.1: The Enigmatic Duo: Estrogen and Progesterone

Let's begin by introducing our enigmatic duo—estrogen and progesterone. These hormones form an essential part of the endocrine orchestra, regulating various physiological processes in the body. While estrogen is often associated with women's reproductive health, progesterone plays a pivotal role during pregnancy, preparing the uterine lining for implantation and supporting early fetal development.

Both hormones are also present in men, although at lower levels, contributing to their overall well-being.

7.2: Estrogen, the Double-Edged Sword

Estrogen, our leading lady in this hormonal narrative, exhibits a dual nature—a nurturing friend and a formidable foe. On one hand, estrogen supports healthy bones, skin, and cognitive function while enhancing mood and overall quality of life. But like all things in life, an excess of estrogen can lead to imbalances, potentially influencing the development of certain cancers, such as breast and ovarian cancer.

7.3: Progesterone, the Balancing Act

Enter progesterone, the balancer of estrogen's power. Progesterone works in harmony with estrogen, mitigating its potential adverse effects. For instance, during the menstrual cycle, it counteracts estrogen's proliferative effects on the uterine lining, ensuring a balanced and healthy environment. However, progesterone's role in breast cancer risk remains a subject of ongoing research and debate.

7.4: The Menopause Dilemma: Hormonal Changes and Cancer Risk

Ah, menopause—a transformative phase that brings with it a myriad of hormonal changes. During menopause, a woman's ovaries produce less estrogen and progesterone, leading to fluctuations that can influence cancer risk. The reduced levels of these hormones may offer some protection against certain cancers, such as uterine cancer, but raise concerns about an increased risk of breast cancer.

7.5: HRT and Cancer Risk: Separating Fact from Fiction

The use of hormone replacement therapy (HRT) to alleviate menopausal symptoms introduces a compelling twist to our tale. HRT involves the administration of estrogen, progesterone (in women with a uterus), or both to balance hormone levels and alleviate menopausal symptoms like hot flashes and mood swings. However, it is crucial to understand the nuanced relationship between HRT and cancer risk.

7.6: The Women's Health Initiative (WHI) Study: A Pivotal Moment

The Women's Health Initiative (WHI) study, a landmark clinical trial, significantly impacted the understanding of HRT's effects on cancer risk. In 2002, the WHI revealed potential associations between HRT and an increased risk of breast cancer, heart disease, and stroke. This revelation led to a decline in HRT usage, causing concern among women seeking relief from menopausal symptoms.

7.7: "I Don't Have a Uterus, Do I Need Progesterone?"

In recent years, bioidentical hormone replacement therapy (BHRT) has emerged as an alternative to traditional HRT. Unlike synthetic hormones, bioidentical hormones possess the same molecular structure as the naturally produced hormones in our bodies. This molecular similarity allows for a smoother integration of hormones and potentially fewer side effects.

Addressing the Uterus Conundrum: "I Don't Have a Uterus, Do I Need Progesterone?"

One of the most common arising questions during HRT discussions is whether women who have had a hysterectomy need progesterone. The answer lies in the delicate balance between estrogen and progesterone. Even women without a uterus may benefit from progesterone to counteract estrogen's potential effects on breast tissue. The decision to include progesterone in HRT should be made individually, with input from a knowledgeable healthcare provider.

Synthetic vs. Natural Hormones: The Plot Thickens

Another pivotal moment in our story is the debate between synthetic and natural hormones. While synthetic hormones have been the traditional go-to for HRT, their molecular differences from endogenous hormones have raised concerns about potential side effects. In contrast, bioidentical hormones offer a promising alternative, providing a more natural approach to hormone replacement.

7.8: The Estrogen Scare: Breast and Ovarian Cancer

Breast and ovarian cancer have long been linked to estrogen exposure. However, the association between hormone replacement therapy and cancer risk is complex. It is essential to remember that individual factors such as genetics, lifestyle choices, and overall health also contribute to cancer risk. Consulting with a healthcare provider to assess personal risk factors is key to making informed decisions about HRT.

In Conclusion: Empowerment through Knowledge

As we conclude this chapter on estrogen and progesterone's intricate connection to cancer risk, I hope you feel empowered with knowledge and a deeper understanding of these hormone's roles in your health. While estrogen and progesterone play significant roles in our well-being, their influence on cancer risk is multifaceted and varies among individuals.

Remember, personalized healthcare guided by expert advice is the key to navigating the hormonal labyrinth. As healthcare professionals, our mission is to help you make informed decisions about your health, ensuring that each choice is tailored to your unique needs.

So, let us embark on this journey together, unraveling the mysteries of estrogen and progesterone and embracing the power of knowledge to promote wellness, vitality, and longevity for all.

8

Testosterone: Empowering Men and Women's Journey – Breaking Barriers: Women and the Testosterone Connection

Once I started experiencing all of the symptoms that I mentioned noticing in previous chapters—mental sluggishness, abdominal weight gain, lack of libido, and more—I had my labs drawn by my hormone specialist only to discover that my testosterone was approximately a third of the amount that I should have in my body. I had the testosterone of a 70-year-old man and didn't even realize it. Right there and then, out of necessity, I embarked on my hormone journey, which to this day continues to fascinate me.

In this enlightening chapter on bioidentical hormones and graceful aging, we embark on a deep exploration of the extraordinary influence of testosterone. Though often stereotyped as a "male hormone," testosterone truthfully, as we shall unveil, is quite a pivotal player in both men's and women's health, impacting vitality, emotional well-being, and relationships—fundamentally shaping the aging process for all.

8.1: The Multifaceted Role of Testosterone

At the heart of the testosterone narrative is its multifaceted role. Often associated solely with male reproductive health, it goes beyond that, impacting essential aspects of aging. It influences the maintenance of muscle mass, bone health, energy levels, and cognitive function—collectively contributing to our overall well-being as we navigate the aging journey.

8.2: Gender-Neutral Vigor: Testosterone for All

Before we delve further, let's discard the misconception that testosterone exclusively pertains to men. Naturally, men produce higher levels of testosterone, but it's just as well a critical hormone for women. In men, it's central to maintaining muscle mass and strength, while in women, it plays an integral role in preserving bone density and overall vitality.

8.3: The Leydig Cells and Adrenals

Understanding the origins of testosterone elucidates its importance. In men, the Leydig cells within the testes primarily produce it. Women's ovaries also contribute, albeit to a lesser extent. Additionally, both genders' adrenal glands produce a small amount of testosterone. This orchestrated production is the bedrock of overall hormone balance, influencing the aging process profoundly.

8.4: Balancing Act: Total vs. Free Testosterone

To comprehend testosterone's impact, we must decipher the difference between total and free testosterone. Total testosterone encompasses hormone bound to proteins, while free testosterone is the unbound and physiologically active form. Striking a balance between these forms is crucial, as they collectively impact energy levels, muscle strength, and overall vitality.

8.5: The Hormonal Tapestry: The Testosterone-Estrogen Ratio

Harmonizing the testosterone-estrogen ratio is pivotal. An imbalance can lead to a plethora of issues, affecting mood, libido, and overall well-being. Optimal balance is attainable through bioidentical hormone therapy; it is the potent tool to ensure this equilibrium and help you cultivate benefits that extend well beyond the physical realm.

8.6: Fueling Desire: Libido's Intimate Link to Testosterone

Often hailed as the ultimate aphrodisiac, testosterone significantly influences libido for both men and women. Balanced testosterone levels elevate sexual desire, breathing new life into relationships and fostering emotional bonds.

8.7: The Emotional Nexus: Testosterone and Mood Enhancement

Testosterone's influence transcends the physical, deeply affecting emotional equilibrium. Optimal levels are associated with stable moods, reduced irritability, and even a decreased risk of depression. Bioidentical testosterone therapy, therefore, can be a vital ally in nurturing emotional well-being and enhancing the ability to navigate life's challenges with resilience.

8.8: Distilling Myth from Reality: Bioidentical Testosterone and Steroids

Let's clarify a common misconception: bioidentical testosterone is not synonymous with illegal steroids. Bioidentical hormones closely mirror the body's natural hormones, offering health benefits without the risks associated with synthetic alternatives.

8.9: Trimming the Waistline: Testosterone's Impact on Body Composition

Testosterone's effects extend to body composition, notably in men. Balanced testosterone levels can lead to reduced abdominal fat, thus not only enhancing physical well-being but also boosting self-esteem and confidence.

8.10: Building Robust Bones: Testosterone's Support for Skeletal Health

Beyond its impact on muscles, testosterone also plays a pivotal role in maintaining bone density. Bone health safeguarding through balanced testosterone levels is crucial in preventing conditions like osteoporosis and reducing the risk of fractures as we age.

8.11: A Strong Heart: Testosterone's Cardiovascular Benefits

Testosterone's benefits go far beyond the physical. Balanced levels contribute to heart health for both men and women. From optimizing cholesterol profiles to enhancing vascular function, testosterone emerges as a guardian against heart disease, promoting longevity.

8.12: The Cognitive Fortifier: Testosterone and Brain Health

Cognitive decline is one of the major concerns as we age, making testosterone's role in brain health paramount. Optimal testosterone levels have been linked to improved memory, focus, and cognitive agility. These benefits extend to the Alzheimer's disease prevention realm, thus solidifying testosterone's role in maintaining cognitive vitality.

8.13: Prostate Harmony: Testosterone's Role in Prostate Health

The notion that testosterone exacerbates prostate issues is a misconception we should put to rest because it doesn't. Contrarily, it actually helps manage them. How, you ask? Well, balanced testosterone levels are associated with a reduced risk of prostate enlargement and cancer, safeguarding prostate health as we age.

8.14: Navigating Andropause: Testosterone, Estrogen, and Progesterone

Much like menopause, men experience andropause— a phase marked by declining hormone levels, including testosterone, estrogen, and progesterone. Each hormone plays a unique role, making their balance crucial for well-being during this transformative phase.

8.15: Embracing Timelessness: Testosterone's Everlasting Influence

Elevating vitality through bioidentical testosterone therapy is an investment in timeless well-being. Its effects span beyond the physical into emotional well-being, infusing confidence and enhancing relationships. Testosterone holds the power to transcend aging, creating a life defined by vibrancy, purpose, and unending enthusiasm.

In Conclusion: Rediscovering Youth through Testosterone

As we thread through the intricate fabric of aging, testosterone emerges as a potent agent of transformation—infusing vitality, enriching relationships, and nurturing emotional resilience.

Bioidentical testosterone therapy becomes a personalized avenue to unlock a life marked by confidence, longevity, and unwavering dynamism. By embracing the multifaceted benefits of testosterone, individuals can shape their aging journey, ensuring it's one rich in vitality, purpose, and enduring zest.

9

Thyroid: The Most Misunderstood Hormone – Mastering the Thyroid's Secrets to Optimal Health

Ever had the feeling that something just wasn't right with your body, but you couldn't put your finger on what was wrong? Was your doctor doing random blood tests on you only to tell you that everything was "normal" even though you knew your body was telling you something? Fear not, friends; I, too, have been there, and we are not alone. Many others have also been in this same untenable predicament. The good news is that there is help, and there are people who can help you. You just need to know where to look.

One early morning, I got to work at the hospital at my usual time, around 6:45 a.m. On that particular day, I had an anesthesia resident working with me in the surgeries as part of her neurosurgery anesthesia training. The resident and I, as usual, went to the preoperative area and met our patient before surgery. After introducing myself and my student to the patient, the patient looked at me and said, "You have a blue aura around you, so I definitely trust you. But you should know that there is something wrong with your thyroid." I had never met this woman in my life, and little did she know that I, too, thought there might be a problem with my thyroid and got my blood tested four days prior to our interaction. I had told no one about the test. So, I'd say this psychic's reading of me was spot on. Despite telling my primary care provider for years that something was wrong with my body, he would constantly dismiss me, telling me that my labwork was "normal." Deep down, I knew something about my body was off, so I had seen a new preventative medicine provider.

Remember in previous chapters where I had mentioned my struggle with gaining weight, losing energy, and constantly feeling tired? Here's where my thyroid journey began.

Thyroid issues often get mixed up with normal signs of aging in people over 50 or 60. Symptoms like tiredness, slower speech, forgetfulness, weight gain, feeling down, hair loss, and feeling cold often get brushed off as just a part of getting older. But actually, these signs are more linked to how your thyroid ages. While doctors might help younger people with these symptoms, they sometimes overlook the same issues in older folks.

As women grow older, they're more likely than men to face thyroid troubles. Because thyroid problems and symptoms of perimenopause or menopause can be quite similar, it can be tricky to diagnose. Even if a woman starts estrogen and progesterone therapy to ease her menopause symptoms, some issues may stick around because of thyroid problems.

For many women, the estrogen and progesterone supplementation approach helps with menopause woes. But if someone still feels down and tired even after getting hormones, that person should have thyroid levels checked. There is importance in getting those levels just right if you want to feel healthy and happy again. Some folks only improve when the thyroid levels are in the upper normal range. When their thyroid levels resume normalcy, the symptoms go away, their health gets better, and they really feel a change. Many healthcare providers, however, do not understand this concept and will dismiss the patient's symptoms when a blood test comes back as "normal."

9.1: Unveiling the Vital Role of the Thyroid: A Master Key to Wellness

Your thyroid plays an integral role in your body's overall functioning. It's a small, butterfly-shaped object in your neck that affects everything in your body—organs, cells, and other hormones. When the thyroid is off, you might end up with high cholesterol, slow thinking, memory issues, weight gain, feeling cold all the time, constipation, changes in your periods, and even skin, hair, and nail changes.

Figuring out that it's the thyroid causing trouble can be difficult because the symptoms can be all over the place. Often, patients get sent from one doctor to another and try all sorts of medications, unaware of the root cause of their problem(s). Symptoms like depression may be treated with antidepressants or weight gain blamed on a bad diet, while the real issue might be a low-functioning thyroid.

Basically, When your thyroid levels are low, it's like your internal engine is slowing down. You may have trouble staying warm and constantly feel tired despite sleeping well. And, while thinning hair, skin, and nails might seem inevitable with aging, the right thyroid treatment can actually improve their state.

9.2: Addressing Mood and Energy: A Closer Look at Thyroid Function

Depression and fatigue often take center stage among the most prevalent symptoms of insufficient thyroid levels. However, these indicators frequently go unnoticed or misdiagnosed due to various factors. The inclination is to attribute mood swings and weariness to the stresses of daily life. Consequently, medical practitioners initiate various treatments, including anti-anxiety medications, antidepressants, and sleep aids, before eventually referring patients to psychiatrists.

Imagine the disappointment patients experience when they realize that their array of medications only exacerbates their condition. Women, in particular, find themselves caught in this cycle, feeling unheard and trapped. In my view, it's essential to consider thyroid deficiency as a potential root cause for symptoms of depression, fatigue, or overall malaise unless proven otherwise. When thyroid levels are optimized, the body is better equipped to manage stressors, and feelings of fatigue and unexplainable mood fluctuations become less common.

Depression, often attributed to a chemical imbalance in the brain, is described by psychiatrists. Yet, given the thyroid's far-reaching influence on metabolism and major organs, it's not surprising that many thyroid patients experience unhappiness and fatigue when their thyroid function is suboptimal. Skin and hair issues, brittle nails, and weight gain can further contribute to feelings of unease and fatigue. Interestingly, research in the New England Journal of Medicine has indicated that natural thyroid preparations, which enhance T3 levels more effectively than T4, often yield better and quicker results.

Many patients express concern that their mental clarity is compromised due to fatigue. A lack of confidence among doctors in supplementing thyroid without substantial blood test results is not uncommon. As a result, many healthcare providers lack the training and experience necessary to optimize thyroid function through natural hormone supplementation (T3 and T4). Dear healthcare provider, please remember it's crucial to focus on the patient's well-being rather than solely relying on numerical values.

It's quite remarkable how thyroid dysfunction is seldom considered when assessing symptoms of depression. Even more astonishing is the tendency to prescribe over-the-counter hormone supplements for detected hypothyroidism that often fail to provide adequate thyroid levels, thereby failing to alleviate symptomatic depression.

9.3: Experiencing Unrelenting Fatigue: A Different Perspective

The struggle becomes a daily ordeal for those who experience persistent fatigue despite adequate sleep. As metabolic rates decrease, so does overall energy. The medical community records an overwhelming number of patient visits related to fatigue, with limited success in finding effective solutions. For many, living with exhaustion has become as commonplace as breathing.

9.4: Thyroid's Role in Cardiovascular Health

The relationship between the heart and the thyroid is intricate. An optimally functioning thyroid helps maintain healthy blood pressure and cholesterol levels, preventing excessive weight gain. While depression, cold intolerance, and skin dryness are well-known thyroid symptoms, other patients face issues like elevated cholesterol, high blood pressure, and hardened arteries.

Numerous studies have highlighted the positive outcomes when patients at risk for heart disease are supplemented with both T4 and T3 thyroid hormones, underscoring thyroid supplementation's significant role in preventive medicine.

9.5: Thyroid Health and Its Impact on Hair

Optimal thyroid supplementation might offer a solution for those battling thinning hair. Most of the time, healthcare providers write off hair loss in females as androgenic hair loss that is age-related.

However, the challenge lies in the fact that 50-year-old women don't possess androgens, making thyroid hormone intervention potentially helpful in preventing hair loss and restoring hair thickness.

9.6: The Connection Between Thyroid and Hair Loss

Hair loss often accompanies thyroid insufficiency, with decreased metabolism in scalp follicles contributing to hair shedding. Brittle hair is also prone to splitting and breakage. T3, a critical hormone for hair maintenance, is often deficient in individuals experiencing hair loss. Those on T4 preparations like Levoxyl or Synthroid may face hair loss, as these medications don't effectively convert T4 to T3.

Many patients have witnessed hair loss reversal with natural thyroid medicine. Paradoxically, one of the side effects of Synthroid is prolonged hair loss.

9.7: Balancing Thyroid Levels for Optimal Well-being

Let's use a lock and key type of theory to explain the phenomenon of thyroid receptor site resistance. As most people know, you need the right key to unlock the correct lock. In this scenario, let's consider your thyroid hormones (TSH, T4, T3) as the key and your thyroid receptor site as the lock. Over time, the lock (thyroid receptor site) starts to get a little rusty, and there either aren't the right kind of keys (TSH, T4, T3) or there aren't enough keys to open every lock. Bioidentical thyroid hormones can work to ensure that there are enough keys for every lock to open those doors and allow you to start feeling like your 20-year-old self again. The following paragraph contains a more scientific explanation of what is in this paragraph.

Low T3 levels or receptor resistance can trigger low thyroid function symptoms even when TSH levels appear normal. Optimal T3 levels or ineffective stimulation of thyroid receptor sites are the primary factors behind the signs and symptoms of hypothyroidism. TSH, often used as an indicator of thyroid function, does not account for low T3 levels or receptor site resistance, rendering it a less-than-ideal diagnostic tool. Replacing thyroid hormones can significantly improve overall health and well-being. However, convincing healthcare providers unfamiliar with natural hormone replacement therapy may pose challenges.

9.8: Selecting the Right Thyroid Hormone

The use of hormones that mirror the body's natural production is crucial to successful hormone replacement. Bioidentical thyroid hormone replacements like Armour Thyroid and compounded natural thyroid preparations have proven effective. A compounded T4 and T3 combination in bioidentical ratios, expertly prepared by a compounding pharmacist, offers better absorption and sustained levels. Pharmaceutical companies promote synthetic forms of hormone replacement, yet they often fall short of adequately converting T4 to T3. Focusing solely on TSH levels neglects the vital roles of free T3 and free T4 at the cellular level.

It's clear that a comprehensive and individualized approach to thyroid supplementation is crucial for achieving optimal well-being.

9.9: Chilled to the Bone: The Mystery of Feeling Cold

Are you someone who is constantly cold and has hands that could sink the Titanic? Sometimes, when your temperature goes too low, your body tries to warm up by making your thyroid work harder. For many women, however, even though their doctor tells them that their thyroid is "okay," they still feel way too cold. Your thyroid and heart are linked. When the thyroid is healthy, it helps control blood pressure, cholesterol, and weight gain. On the other hand, when the thyroid is not working right, you could have higher cholesterol and blood pressure and trouble with your arteries.

9.10: Hair Today, Gone Tomorrow

The thyroid also has a role in how your hair looks. If your thyroid is off, your hair can thin and break. But the hormone T3 can help keep your hair healthy. Even so, many women who take thyroid medicine still struggle with hair loss because their medication doesn't give them enough T3. Yet another reason to switch to bioidentical, natural thyroid medication—are you keeping count?

Even if your TSH levels seem normal, if your T3 is low or your thyroid isn't responding well, you could still feel tired and low. TSH is like a messenger that tells the thyroid to make more hormones. But it neither notices when T3 levels are off nor when the thyroid isn't responding well. For this reason, it's important to find a healthcare provider who gets this concept and can help with natural thyroid hormones.

9.11: What Thyroid Medication Should I be Using?

When it comes down to deciding which thyroid medicine to take, natural options like Armour Thyroid and natural Thyroid medications are better because they match what your body makes. They are natural bioidentical medication options made by a special compounding pharmacist that contain both T4 and T3 in the right amounts. Other medicines like Synthroid or levothyroxine only have T4, but it doesn't always change into enough T3. While these drugs might keep TSH and T4 normal, many people still feel low because they lack enough T3.

Some doctors only look at TSH, but that's not enough. The most important levels are free T3 and free T4. T3 really matters for your cells, so that's where the focus should be. While we're taught that

T4 changes into T3 as needed, that's not always true, especially as we age. Many women over 50 have lower T3 levels, and our bodies convert less T4 into T3.

The widely recognized thyroid medications in the current market include products such as Synthroid or Levoxyl. These formulations solely comprise T4, with the presumption that T4 will transform into active T3. Pharmaceutical companies assert that these conventional synthetic versions offer a consistent and controlled hormonal balance. However, my findings challenge this assumption, revealing that T4 and Synthroid do not readily convert into T3. Despite maintaining normal TSH and T4 levels, many patients still report classic symptoms of low thyroid function. If physicians were to assess the free T3 levels in these patients, they would be surprised to discover that a majority are notably low.

Healthcare practitioners have traditionally concentrated solely on TSH levels, inadvertently overlooking the critical indicators: free T3 and free T4. T3 plays a vital role at the cellular level, warranting our focus on achieving optimal T3 levels. Additionally, the conventional healthcare understanding dictates that only T4 needs replacement, as the body should automatically convert T4 to T3. However, reality doesn't align with this notion. As we age, the body produces decreasing amounts of T3. Subsequently, a significant proportion of women over 50 will exhibit lower-than-normal free T3 levels as the conversion of T4 to T3 diminishes over time.

Natural thyroid has been used for a long time, even since 1892. It can be a powerful way to help people feel better when their thyroid is not working as it should.

10

Melatonin: The Aging Loophole – Sleep, Rejuvenate, Repeat: Melatonin's Ageless Magic

Aging doesn't need to be as challenging as commonly perceived; the way you see the older people in your life aging like milk doesn't have to be you. Melatonin, a naturally occurring sleep aid and an integral component of the longevity equation, has been a catalyst in shaping healthcare providers' perspectives on the prospect of effectively thwarting age-related ailments.

Scientific evidence validated by studies on animals sharing genetic traits with humans has unveiled that melatonin possesses the potential to decelerate the aging process. This revelation suggests that melatonin's benefits extend to us as well. Moreover, given the robust findings from these investigations, researchers are now exploring melatonin's potential as a potent antioxidant, cancer inhibitor, and immune system enhancer. They are also exploring its positive effects on conditions such as heart disease, AIDS, Alzheimer's disease, and Parkinson's disease. Current research underscores melatonin's extensive potential for both immediate and long-term advantages.

Melatonin originates from a series of biochemical events that commence with the amino acid tryptophan. Tryptophan transforms into serotonin, which is then, catalyzed into melatonin through enzymatic action. Following its release by the pineal gland, melatonin enters the local bloodstream and eventually reaches the body's circulation, offering access to every bodily fluid and tissue. Its production is predominantly influenced by the night and day cycle; in the presence of light, melatonin production decreases, while in darkness, melatonin levels surge, inducing drowsiness.

Unlike most hormones, melatonin does not always necessitate a receptor site. The compact molecular structure and solubility of melatonin enable it to permeate nearly every cell in the body. Consequently, melatonin seems to exert influence on various organs and systems, extending beyond its role as a natural tranquilizer.

With over five decades of research supporting its safety across multiple clinical applications, melatonin plays a pivotal role in our sleep patterns as it decreases with age. Any disruption in sleep quality or the loss of deep sleep stages negatively impacts the immune system and overall well-being. Maintaining optimal melatonin levels is essential to mitigate numerous age-related conditions. Most significantly, recent medical research underscores melatonin's crucial role in both cancer prevention and treatment.

Like other hormones, melatonin cannot halt the passage of time, yet it can mitigate many of time's debilitating effects. By boosting immune function, melatonin guides us towards healthier aging. Sleep—often regarded as nature's remedy—possesses regenerative power that can effectively repair damage incurred during waking hours. The restorative phase of deep sleep, particularly stage 4 sleep, is facilitated by melatonin's ebbs and flows. Melatonin levels rise substantially at night, peaking around 2:00 a.m., enhancing the body and mind's recovery from daily stresses.

As age progresses, melatonin production declines, leading to insomnia and sleep disorders. Sleepless nights significantly hamper the immune system and overall disposition. Travelers have found employing melatonin to combat jet lag effective because by consuming melatonin upon arriving in a new time zone, the circadian rhythm adjusts more swiftly. Unlike prescription sleep aids with adverse side effects and addictive potential, melatonin is a safe, potent, and non-addictive hormone.

10.1: Maintaining Immune Vigor

The correlation between the absence of melatonin and immune system decline is evident. Studies involving animals have consistently demonstrated that when the pineal gland is removed, hindering melatonin synthesis, subjects experience a form of immunosuppression. However, the oral restoration of melatonin triggers the revival of a robust immune system.

Beyond its role as an immune system enhancer, melatonin is acclaimed as a formidable antioxidant. A study conducted in 2001 showcased melatonin's remarkable ability to scavenge free radicals, potentially benefiting both mind and body. Antioxidants are vital in combating free radicals (the unstable molecules that attack stable molecules to obtain the missing electron). While the lifespan of a free radical is brief, its damage can be long-lasting. Some medical experts believe that free radicals are the root cause of aging, as they disrupt functioning atoms, leading to cellular degradation.

Melatonin's anti-oxidative prowess is particularly noteworthy in countering conditions linked to oxidative stress, such as Alzheimer's disease, cancer, Parkinson's disease, multiple sclerosis, and rheumatoid arthritis.

10.2: Facing the Challenge of Cancer

Because melatonin bolsters the immune response and combats free radicals, its potential as a tumor growth inhibitor is logical. Research has illuminated melatonin's indirect attack on breast cancer cells and its ability to impede the progression of prostate cancer cells.

Closing Chapter
Embracing the Future of Wellness with Bioidentical Hormones

I am filled with a profound sense of hope and optimism as I stand at the threshold of concluding this exploration into the realm of bioidentical hormones. Throughout this journey, we've delved deep into bioidentical hormones' science, history, and practical applications. And while at it, uncovered the tremendous potential they hold for our overall health and well-being. The transformative possibilities of bioidentical hormones have reaffirmed my commitment as a medical professional to keep empowering individuals with the knowledge and tools to make informed decisions about their health.

In this closing chapter, I want to reflect on some key takeaways and offer a glimpse into the future of wellness with bioidentical hormones. We've seen that these hormones closely mimic those produced by our own bodies and have the power to restore balance, giving you a renewed sense of vitality. But the journey doesn't end here; it's merely the beginning of a new era in personalized medicine and holistic well-being.

A Journey of Self-Discovery

The exploration of bioidentical hormones has been, in essence, a journey of self-discovery. It has led us to reevaluate the conventional hormone therapy approaches and prompted us to consider a more natural, individualized, and patient-centered paradigm. We've learned that hormonal imbalances can manifest in various ways, affecting not only our physical health but also our emotional and mental health.

The Power of Precision Medicine

Bioidentical hormones epitomize the concept of precision medicine. They allow us to tailor treatment plans to the unique needs of each individual, recognizing that one size does not fit all when it comes to hormone therapy. This personalized approach ensures that we optimize outcomes while minimizing risks and side effects.

Empowering Patients

Education has been a central theme of this journey. It's crucial to empower patients with the knowledge they need to make informed decisions about their health. By understanding their hormonal imbalances and treatment options, individuals can actively participate in their care and take control of their well being.

Holistic Well-Being

Bioidentical hormones also invite us to embrace a more holistic view of health. They remind us that our bodies are interconnected systems, and as such, achieving optimal health requires addressing not just hormonal imbalances but also factors such as nutrition, exercise, stress management, and sleep.

Looking Ahead

As we look to the future, the possibilities are exciting and promising. Research into bioidentical hormones continues to expand, offering hope for improved treatments, reduced risks, and enhanced therapeutic outcomes. The integration of bioidentical hormones into mainstream medicine is gaining momentum, fostering collaboration between conventional and integrative healthcare practitioners.

In closing, I'd like to express my gratitude to you for accompanying me on this journey through the fascinating world of bioidentical hormones. My fervent hope as a medical professional is that this book has provided you with a comprehensive understanding of these remarkable hormones and their potential to transform lives. Let us continue to explore, innovate, and collaborate in the pursuit of optimal health and wellness for all.

The future of wellness with bioidentical hormones is bright, and together, we can usher in an era of personalized, holistic, and empowered healthcare. Thank you for being a part of this important conversation, and may your path to well-being be guided by knowledge, compassion, and the pursuit of a healthier, happier life.

www.ingramcontent.com/pod-product-compliance
Lightning Source LLC
Chambersburg PA
CBHW070955250726
48663CB00002B/235